Cognitive behavioural therapy

An information guide

Neil A. Rector, PhD, CPsych

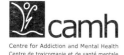

camh

Centre for Addiction and Mental Health
Centre de toxicomanie et de santé mentale

A Pan American Health Organization /
World Health Organization Collaborating Centre

Library and Archives Canada Cataloguing in Publication
Rector, Neil A.
    Cognitive-behavioural therapy : an information guide / Neil Rector.
Issued also in French under title: Thérapie cognitivo-comportementale.
Includes bibliographical references.
Issued also in electronic formats.
ISBN 978-1-77052-294-7
    1. Cognitive therapy. I. Centre for Addiction and Mental Health II. Title.
RC489.C63R43 2010   616.89'142   C2010-904213-1

ISBN: 978-1-77052-294- 7 (PRINT)
ISBN: 978-1-77052-295-4 (PDF)
ISBN: 978-1-77052-296-1 (HTML)
ISBN: 978-1-77052-297-8 (EPUB)

PM087

Printed in Canada

This publication may be available in other formats. For information about alternate
formats or other CAMH publications, or to place an order, please contact Sales and
Distribution:
Toll-free: 1 800 661-1111
Toronto: 416 595-6059
E-mail: publications@camh.net
Online store: http://store.camh.net
Website: www.camh.net

Disponible en français sous le titre :
Thérapie cognitivo-comportementale : Guide d'Information

This guide was produced by the following:
Development: Michelle Maynes, CAMH
Editorial: Diana Ballon, Jacquelyn Waller-Vintar, CAMH
Graphic design: Nancy Leung, Mara Korkola, CAMH
Print production: Christine Harris, CAMH

3973c / 11-2010 / PM087

CONTENTS

About the author

Neil A. Rector, PhD, CPsych, is a clinical psychologist and research scientist at Sunnybrook Health Sciences Centre in Toronto. He is a founding fellow of the Academy of Cognitive Therapy (USA) and is an active clinician, educator and researcher in the area of cognitive-behavioural therapy. Dr. Rector is also the author of two other information guides in this series: *Anxiety Disorders* and *Obsessive-Compulsive Disorder*.

Acknowledgments

Thanks to the many people who reviewed and commented on earlier drafts of this guide. Reviewers included Diana Ballon, Eva Dipoce, Lori Douglas, Alexander Rosenfield and Krystyna Walko. Professional reviewers included Lance Hawley, PhD, CPsych, Judith Laposa, PhD, CPsych, and Sandra L. Mendlowitz, PhD, CPsych.

Introduction

This information guide is for people who may be considering or currently participating in cognitive-behavioural therapy (CBT) as a treatment, either alone or with medications or another form of psychotherapy. The guide is also for people who want to better understand CBT to help them support a family member or friend.

The aim of this guide is to provide an easy-to-read introduction to a rich and complex therapy. The guide describes the nature and process of CBT—what it is and what it involves. It also outlines the goals of CBT and the tasks used in therapy to help people reach those goals. For a better understanding of the many aspects of this form of psychotherapy, the guide should be read from cover to cover; however, some readers may prefer to dip into parts of the book that are of particular interest.

Details in the examples in this guide have been altered to protect client anonymity.

1 What is cognitive-behavioural therapy?

For much of the 20th century, the dominant form of psychotherapy was psychoanalysis. This approach involved seeing a therapist several times a week, often for years. Then, in the 1970s, an explosion of different approaches to psychotherapy began to appear. Many of these were short term, lasting only weeks or months.

In 1979, *Time* magazine reported that there were almost 200 different types of psychotherapy. As of 2010, there are thought to be between 400 and 500 types. However, when directly compared, only a handful of therapy approaches have been shown to be highly effective for the kinds of problems people usually seek help for, such as depression, anxiety, phobias and stress-related problems. Of the many therapies available, *cognitive-behavioural therapy* (CBT) is increasingly identified as the "gold standard"—that is, the best type of therapy for these difficulties. This conclusion is supported by more than 375 clinical trial studies since 1977 and also by current international treatment guidelines, which are based on the collective knowledge of experts in the field. For instance, the National Institute of Mental Health (NIMH) in the United States and the National Institute for Health and Clinical Excellence (NICE) in the United Kingdom have concluded that among the available psychological treatments for anxiety and depression, CBT is recommended as the first-line psychological treatment.

CBT has been shown to be effective for people of all ages, from early childhood to older adults, and for people of different levels of education and income and various cultural backgrounds. It has also been shown to be effective when used in individual or group formats.

Introducing CBT

CBT is an intensive, short-term (six to 20 sessions), problem-oriented approach. It was designed to be quick, practical and goal-oriented and to provide people with long-term skills to keep them healthy.

The focus of CBT is on the here-and-now—on the problems that come up in a person's day-to-day life. CBT helps people to look at how they interpret and evaluate what is happening around them and the effects these perceptions have on their emotional experience.

Childhood experiences and events, while not the focus of CBT, may also be reviewed. This review can help people to understand and address emotional upset that emerged early in life, and to learn how these experiences may influence current responses to events.

According to CBT, the way people feel is linked to the way they think about a situation and not simply to the nature of the situation itself. This idea is rooted in ancient Eastern and Western philosophies and became part of a mainstream psychotherapy approach in the early 1960s. Aaron T. Beck, the father of CBT, described the negative thinking patterns associated with depression (i.e., critical thoughts about oneself, the world and the future) in his early writings. He also outlined ways to target and reduce negative thoughts as a way to improve mood. In later work, Beck and his colleagues focused on the content and processes of thought related to anxiety and ways to treat anxiety problems. Since its creation, CBT has expanded into one of the most widely used therapeutic approaches.

What happens in CBT?

In CBT, you learn to identify, question and change the thoughts, attitudes, beliefs and assumptions related to your problematic emotional and behavioural reactions to certain kinds of situations.

By monitoring and recording your thoughts during situations that lead to emotional upset, you learn that the way you think can contribute to emotional problems such as depression and anxiety. In CBT, you learn to reduce these emotional problems by:

• identifying distortions in your thinking
• seeing thoughts as ideas about what is going on rather than as facts
• "standing back" from your thinking to consider situations from different viewpoints.

For CBT to be effective, you must be open and willing to discuss your thoughts, beliefs and behaviours and to participate in exercises during sessions. For best results, you must also be willing to do homework between sessions.

What conditions can CBT treat?

CBT is an effective treatment for many psychological conditions. These include:

- mood disorders, such as depression and bipolar disorder
- anxiety disorders, including specific phobias (e.g., fear of animals, heights, enclosed spaces), panic disorder, social phobia (social anxiety disorder), generalized anxiety disorder, obsessive-compulsive disorder and posttraumatic stress disorder
- bulimia nervosa and binge eating disorder
- body dysmorphic disorder (i.e., body image)
- substance use disorders (i.e., smoking, alcohol and other drugs).

CBT can also be used to help people with:

- psychosis
- habits such as hair pulling, skin picking and tics
- sexual and relationship problems
- insomnia
- chronic fatigue syndrome
- chronic (persistent) pain
- long-standing interpersonal problems.

A similar framework is used to treat different emotional problems in CBT; however, the approach and strategies vary and are tailored to address each specific problem.

Why is CBT an effective therapy?

CBT is an effective therapeutic approach because it:

- is structured
- is problem-focused and goal-oriented
- teaches proven strategies and skills
- emphasizes the importance of a good, collaborative therapeutic relationship between the therapist and client.

In describing how CBT works, the focus of this guide will be on how it applies to treating people experiencing emotional distress.

2 The basics of cognitive-behavioural therapy

Most often, people think of their distress as emerging directly from events and situations in their lives: "I had an argument with my partner this morning and I am still angry," "My boss criticized my work and I feel so defeated" or "I read the business section of the paper this morning, saw that my stock was down, and felt very anxious." In each example, the person highlights how the situation has *caused* his or her emotional upset.

SITUATION 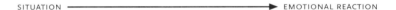 EMOTIONAL REACTION

However, what you feel in response to a situation is determined not only by the situation, but also by the way you *perceive* the situation or make meaning of it. This way of seeing your emotional reaction as determined by what you think about a situation is a basic assumption of the cognitive-behavioural approach.

For example, if you are fast asleep at 3:00 a.m. and you are woken by a crashing sound at your bedroom window, the way you respond to the situation will differ, depending on what you think is happening. If you think it is an intruder, you are likely to feel fear and terror and respond by rushing out of the room to safety. If you think that it must be your roommate (assuming you have one) coming in through the window because he or she has forgotten the key (again!), you will likely feel frustration and annoyance and respond by arguing with your roommate. Finally, if you think it may be your romantic partner coming over for a late night rendezvous, you will likely feel and act with excitement.

The nature of automatic thoughts

In each previous example, the event is the same: a loud noise at the window at 3:00 a.m. However, you could have a different, quick thought to evaluate the situation, or what is referred to in CBT as an *automatic thought*—a thought that "pops" into your mind and shapes the particular emotion experienced (e.g., fear, annoyance, excitement) and the resulting behaviour (e.g., escape, confrontation, warm greeting).

More than the situation itself, it is these pop-up, automatic thoughts that lead to your emotional and behavioural reactions.

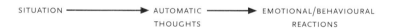

SITUATION ──────────▶ AUTOMATIC ──────────▶ EMOTIONAL/BEHAVIOURAL
                      THOUGHTS   REACTIONS

Evaluating automatic thoughts

Automatic thoughts are usually so brief and quickly overridden by your awareness of the emotions that follow from them that you may not even notice them.

The ability to notice and evaluate your automatic thoughts when you are in the midst of upsetting situations is one of the core skills learned and practiced in CBT. In CBT, you learn to ask yourself,

"What was going through my mind when I noticed feeling emotionally upset?"

Try this CBT exercise now: Think of a time earlier in the day or in the past couple of days when you felt some kind of emotional upset, such as anxiety, sadness or anger. Now, try to remember what you were thinking about at the time. As you recall your thoughts during this event, you may become more aware of automatic thoughts that were going through your mind that you had not noticed at the time.

Identifying your automatic thoughts helps you to clarify the nature of the resulting emotion and understand why the situation was so upsetting.

Patterns in automatic thoughts

When people begin to monitor and record their automatic thoughts, they often recognize a *pattern*. In his earliest writings on CBT in the 1960s, Aaron T. Beck found that patients who were depressed often reported having automatic thoughts characterized by negative perceptions of themselves ("I'm worthless"), of the world around them ("Nobody likes me"), and of the future ("I'm hopeless and can't change"). This pattern of thinking was termed the "cognitive triad" of depression.

Beck's later writings from the 1980s described a pattern of automatic thoughts that seemed to be more uniquely related to anxiety, with clients reporting more thoughts related to threat and danger ("What if something terrible happens?") and the inability to cope ("I'm overwhelmed, I can't go on like this").

While everyone has their own way of seeing situations and events in their lives, when people experience depression or anxiety the content of their automatic thoughts begins to take on a predictable and characteristic form.

A goal of CBT is to help you become aware of your automatic thoughts and to learn to stand back and question, evaluate and correct inaccurate, negative automatic thoughts. However, CBT is *not* trying to teach positive thinking as a solution to life's problems. Rather, the goal is for you to learn to evaluate your experiences and problems from different perspectives—positive, negative and neutral—to arrive at accurate conclusions and creative solutions to your difficulties.

Identifying distortions in automatic thoughts

A second feature of negative automatic thoughts in people with emotional distress is that they tend to reflect *distortions* or errors in thinking. For example, the person who thinks that "I will never find a partner" because of one unsuccessful date is *catastrophizing* the outcome of this date and is more likely to experience excessive emotional upset than the person who thinks "This date didn't go well but hopefully things will go better next time." In another example, a student who concludes that a low mark on a recent exam means that he is "stupid" and a "failure" is *labelling* himself and thinking in *all-or-nothing* terms, and is more likely to be distressed than a student who thinks, "I didn't do as well as I would have liked but I'll seek out extra help and study harder next time."

Distortions in thinking exaggerate the emotional significance of common, everyday events. One aim of CBT is to help you become more aware of distortions in your perception of day-to-day experiences, especially when you are very upset.

Everyone has negative automatic thoughts that pop up in the flow of consciousness, and most of us have cognitive distortions from time to time. However, some people are more likely to have automatic thoughts related to depression and anxiety, and to have more cognitive distortions. The CBT approach suggests that automatic thoughts are influenced by two "deeper" levels of thinking, which can make people more vulnerable to having recurrent negative and distorted thinking patterns. These deeper levels are known as *rules and assumptions* and *core beliefs*.

Rules and assumptions

From early childhood, you learn certain rules and assumptions through your interactions with family members and the world around you. For instance, you may learn rules about:

- how to relate with others (e.g., "If you don't have anything nice to say, then don't say anything at all")
- the acceptability of expressing emotions (e.g., "Don't ever let them see you sweat")
- your performance (e.g., "If you can't do something perfectly, then it's not even worth trying" or "I should be great at everything I do").

These rules and assumptions may not be obvious to you and remain out of your awareness. However, when you begin to monitor your automatic thoughts in upsetting situations, you become aware of patterns in your automatic thoughts that are linked to your underlying rules and assumptions.

For example, if you hold an underlying assumption that you must be the best at everything you do, you are more likely to be distressed by a less than optimal outcome (e.g., failed test, lost promotion, unsuccessful job interview) than someone who does not hold this assumption.

Automatic thoughts can arise from underlying rules and assumptions.

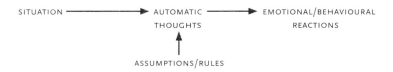

CBT aims to help you become more aware of your own rules and assumptions and how these contribute to a pattern of negative automatic thoughts in emotionally upsetting situations.

Core beliefs

At the deepest level of cognition, even deeper than your rules and assumptions, are your *core beliefs*. Core beliefs usually develop early in life. They reflect rigid and absolute notions about yourself, others and the world. Examples of positive core beliefs are "I'm attractive," "I'm smart" and "I'm loveable." Examples of negative core beliefs are "I'm worthless" or "I'm weak"; "others are danger-ous" and "not to be trusted"; and "the world is a scary place" and "overwhelming."

Aaron T. Beck suggested that people with negative core beliefs are more at risk of developing depression or anxiety than people with positive core beliefs. Negative core beliefs may be inactive and not affect a person's life until a stressful life event, such as a death in the family, a break-up or job loss activates these beliefs. For example, a woman who has a core belief that she is "unlovable" may also believe that if she works hard to please her partner, he may love her anyway. However, if her partner breaks up with her, her core belief of being "unlovable" may be reactivated, and increase her vulnerability to depression or anxiety.

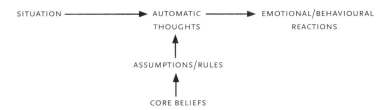

A basic assumption of CBT is that people can learn to identify, evaluate and change their assumptions and core beliefs, just as they are able to identify and change their negative automatic thoughts. When you begin to reduce negative assumptions and beliefs, you also begin to have fewer negative and distorted automatic thoughts. Reducing the negative underlying assumptions and core beliefs that give rise to your emotional problems lessens your emotional upset and also offers you some protection from becoming depressed and anxious again.

In summary, CBT is different from many other therapeutic approaches because it focuses on helping you learn to identify the relationship between your thoughts, feelings and behaviours. While each of these are interdependent (they all serve to influence each other), CBT gives special attention to the role of cognition (automatic thoughts, rules and assumptions and core beliefs) in creating and maintaining emotional difficulties such as depression and anxiety.

CBT aims to help you identify, evaluate and change your habitual thinking patterns at each of these levels of cognition. Working with the therapist, you learn that assigning less extreme, more helpful and more accurate meanings to negative events leads to less extreme and less disturbing emotional and behavioural responses. Once you have learned these skills in therapy, you will become your own therapist, with the ability to manage difficult experiences and emotional upset on your own.

3 CBT approaches to cognitive change

Automatic thoughts pop up all the time in everyone's minds. Some of these thoughts are positive, some are neutral and some are negative. The ones that are of particular interest in CBT are the negative automatic thoughts that relate to periods of intense moods. An early aim of CBT is to help you learn to identify negative automatic thoughts and cognitive distortions in problematic situations. This skill can be learned relatively quickly by some people, while for others it will take practice and require patience.

Identifying relations between thoughts, moods and behaviours

The first step toward identifying automatic thoughts and cognitive distortions in problematic situations is for you to discuss recent upsetting situations with your CBT therapist. This discussion helps you to learn about the relationship between your thoughts, moods and behaviours, as in the following example:

> *Therapist: Can you think of a situation in the past week when you felt upset?*

Peter: I was sitting on the subway and noticing all of the couples together.

Therapist: And what feelings came up for you as you were noticing the couples?

Peter: I was feeling sad and angry.

Therapist: And what were you thinking about as you were feeling sad and angry?

Peter: I was thinking everyone seems to have someone in their life but me, and it's just not fair.

Therapist: And if it's true that everyone seems to have someone but you, do you think this says something about you?

Peter: Yah, that I'm a loser and will always be alone.

Therapist: And what did you do when you were thinking and feeling this way?

Peter: After a while I couldn't take it anymore so I got off the subway even though I hadn't reached my stop yet. I went home and just sat on my bed thinking about all of this.

In this example, the following elements are identified:

Situation: On the subway, noticing couples
Moods: Sad and angry
Thoughts: Everyone has someone but me, it isn't fair, I'm a loser, I will be alone forever.
Behaviours: Escape from subway, return home to ruminate

This example shows that to understand why Peter was feeling sad and angry, we need to understand what he was thinking:

- that he does not have a relationship and really wants to be in one
- that it does not seem fair to him that everyone else seems to get what he desires so much in his life
- that because he does not have someone now, he will never find someone and will always be alone.

As an exercise, try to think of a situation in the past week that was upsetting. Please take a moment to see if you can identify the following:

Situation: _____
(Where were you? Were you with anyone?)

Moods: _____
(What were you feeling?)

Thoughts: _____
(What was going through your mind?)

Behaviours:_____
(What did you do? How did you cope?)

Questioning and evaluating negative automatic thoughts

As you learn to identify your negative automatic thoughts, you will also learn to question and evaluate these thoughts. A main goal of CBT is to help you learn to see your thoughts as ideas that do not necessarily reflect reality. In other words, just because you think something does not always mean it is true.

To help you move toward this goal, the therapist will direct you through "cognitive restructuring" exercises. In these exercises, you will learn to stand back and question your negative automatic thoughts and to evaluate the evidence that either supports or does not support the thoughts. You will then be able to draw conclusions about the accuracy of your thoughts.

A CBT therapist working with Peter in the previous example might ask him the following questions:

- "Do you know anyone that you like and respect who is not currently in a relationship?"
- "Do you have any past experiences in romantic relationships?"
- "If you had a good friend that had the same thoughts about himself or herself, what would you say to that friend?"
- "Are you possibly discounting any life experiences to suggest that you will not be completely alone?"
- "Are you potentially blaming yourself for something that you do not have complete control of?"

The goal here is not to challenge Peter's thinking but rather to move him to a questioning mode and to consider the accuracy of his automatic thoughts based on evidence from his life.

Identifying and correcting cognitive distortions

Identifying and changing negative automatic thoughts related to strong feelings also involves learning to identify distortions or "errors" in thinking as you experience or recall upsetting situations.

Distortions in thinking are more likely to occur when you feel distressed. This is because emotional distress can wear you down, and feeling worn down tends to make people more reliant on shortcuts or more simplistic ways of thinking. Everyone has distortions in thinking at times. Below are some types of distortions in thinking (Burns, 1999), with examples to illustrate what they look like:

- *All-or-nothing (black-and-white) thinking*: When you see things as either black or white with no grey area in between (e.g., Amina finished the term with three A+s, two As and one B+ and is thinking that because she did not ace all her courses she is a "failure").
- *Disqualifying the positive*: When you discount positive experiences and continue to focus only on the negative (e.g., Josh is a devoted father who helps his son with homework every night and spends as much time with him as possible on the weekends. Recent business travel has kept him away from home more than usual, leading him to conclude that he is a "lousy father").
- *Overgeneralization*: When you see a single event as something that will never end (e.g., Ingrid felt anxious in the meeting at work and now concludes that she will never be able to interact with her colleagues comfortably).
- *Mental filter*: When you pay attention to a small negative detail in an experience so that it takes on great importance (e.g., Dwight is speaking to a group of 10 youth at his church and continually focuses his attention on one person who seems disinterested in what he has to say rather than the other nine who seem quite engaged).
- *Catastrophizing*: When you think of the worst case scenario—that is, you assume that a situation will be more awful or horrible than it is likely to be (e.g., Susan awakes one morning and notices a rash on the back of her leg. Rather than thinking of all the factors that could have contributed to the rash, she quickly concludes that she has skin cancer and rushes to the doctor).

- *Mind reading*: When you jump to conclusions thinking that some-one is thinking of you negatively before you have all of the facts (e.g., Guy walks into a movie theatre and as he goes to sit down, he trips and stumbles and spills his popcorn and drink. He thinks that everyone must be thinking that "he's a total loser").
- *Personalization*: When you see events not going well as a result of something about you (e.g., Charmaine is hosting a party and sees that two guests are sitting quietly on their own. She begins to think it must be her fault that they are not having a good time).

Recording your thoughts

Early in treatment, the CBT therapist will question you in ways that help you to identify and question your negative automatic thoughts and cognitive distortions. As you progress, the therapist will ask you to use the *thought record* between sessions as homework. With practice, you will become skilled at using the thought record to re-cord, question and evaluate your automatic thoughts and to reduce emotional distress in your day-to-day life.

The best time to do the thought record is soon after the situation or event that causes distress. This is when you are most aware of the thoughts related to your experience. However, sometimes this is difficult; for instance, if the problem comes up at work or at other times where it would be inconvenient or where your privacy would be compromised. When this is the case, try to find a time later the same day to record the details, before they fade, and to help you feel better about the situation sooner, rather than later.

The first three columns of the thought record (shown in Table 1) are used to record the situation that you were in when you began to experience a strong emotion, the automatic thoughts related to the event or experience, and the strength of your emotional reaction.

The example in Table 1 shows how a client named Nancy reported on the experience of anxiety when thinking about an upcoming event:

Table 1. The thought record: Example

SITUATION	AUTOMATIC THOUGHTS	EMOTIONS
Thinking about driving up north to the cottage	I am going to have a panic attack while driving Everyone will be angry with me I won't be able to cope with the situation	Fear (80%)

Once Nancy listed her automatic thoughts, the next step was for her to consider the evidence that supported and did not support her thoughts and to evaluate their accuracy, as shown in Table 2.

Table 2. Evaluating the evidence

EVIDENCE FOR:	EVIDENCE AGAINST:
Felt nervous on the drive up north last time.	Even though I felt nervous, I did not have a full-fledged panic attack.
People did seem somewhat put off by the fact that I spent my night resting in my room after the drive last time.	Even though I was uncomfortable, I was still able to drive and I got us there safely.

EVIDENCE FOR:	EVIDENCE AGAINST:
	My boyfriend will be driving with me and he is very understanding and supportive and won't get angry with me.
	I have travelled five other times this year without any anxiety at all.
	Even if I do get very anxious and have a panic attack, I know that it is not dangerous to me. I will cope by trying not to catastrophize the anxiety.

By evaluating the evidence supporting or not supporting the negative automatic thoughts, both through discussion with her therapist and through the use of the thought record, Nancy was able to arrive at a more balanced alternative appraisal of the situation. As is often the case for everyone, just a little bit of new information led Nancy to a different and less upsetting interpretation of the situation.

Targeting assumptions and beliefs

As therapy progresses, the CBT therapist will introduce other cognitive strategies and homework worksheets to target your underlying assumptions and core beliefs.

One way to identify your core beliefs and assumptions is to use your thought records to identify specific situations that lead to emotional distress, and to look for themes that recur. The CBT therapist can then help you to question and evaluate these assumptions and beliefs and to generate less distressing, alternative viewpoints as they occur in upsetting situations.

Another way assumptions and beliefs are targeted for change in CBT is to write down a negative core belief on one side of the page, for example, "unlikeable" and an alternative, less distressing belief that you would prefer to hold about yourself, for example, "likeable" on the other side of the page. You would then be asked to keep track of your experiences over the week, noting instances where the negative or positive belief seemed to be supported. In situations where you collected evidence to support the negative belief, you would also be asked to review the situation carefully for supporting and contrary evidence to arrive at a more balanced perspective.

BEHAVIOURAL EXPERIMENTS

A powerful tool for questioning and evaluating underlying assumptions and core beliefs is to test their validity with behavioural experiments. For instance, if you had an underlying assumption that "If I make a mistake everyone will laugh and ridicule me," you might be asked to perform an experiment to determine what actually happens when mistakes are made. Of course, you will only conduct experiments that you think you are ready for, and after you have developed strategies to cope with the full range of possible outcomes from these types of experiments.

When you are ready, you may, for example, be asked to make a mistake on purpose, such as to go into a store and drop change while in line, or to spill a drink in a cafeteria. This will allow you to see the extent to which: a) people notice, b) people respond (e.g., do others laugh and ridicule you as feared or alternatively, do people not seem to notice or criticize you), and c) how well you can cope with the situation.

In summary, the initial focus of CBT is to help you identify and change negative automatic thoughts that lead to emotional distress in problematic situations. You learn skills to identify and correct negative automatic thoughts and the cognitive distortions that fuel strong moods. The main tool for cognitive change is the thought record. Other cognitive strategies are used to consolidate progress with changing negative automatic thoughts and the deeper assumptions and beliefs. These include:

• examining the advantages and disadvantages of holding such beliefs
• examining the evidence that supports and does not support the assumptions and beliefs
• trying to find less extreme, more middle-ground views of oneself, others and the world
• performing behavioural experiments.

4 CBT approaches to behavioural change

So far, we have focused on the "C" of CBT, which refers to changing the cognitive aspects, or thinking, that can lead to emotional distress. We now move on to the "B" in CBT, which refers to changing the behaviours that can worsen and prolong negative moods.

Changes in thinking and behaviours go hand in hand: When you change the way you think about a situation or problem, your behaviours may also change. The reverse is also true: When you change how you approach a situation or problem, you may come to think differently about it. For instance, if you smoke, and some new information leads you to believe that smoking is more dangerous to your health than you once thought, this may lead you to quit smoking (i.e., cognitive change leads to behavioural change). Or, to turn it around, if you go for a week without smoking because you are sick or unable to smoke, it could lead you to think, "If I can go a week without smoking, maybe I could go a month." This thinking could lead to a new behavioural goal of trying to quit smoking for a month (i.e., behavioural change leads to cognitive change).

CBT uses a variety of behavioural methods and strategies to reduce your distress, which are introduced on the following pages.

Self-monitoring

Chapter 3 outlined the use of thought records to identify and evaluate negative thoughts and cognitive distortions. Thought records are one type of self-monitoring strategy that you will be asked to do in CBT. You may also be asked to do other forms of self-monitoring, such as:

- monitoring your moods or feelings of pleasure or mastery day by day, perhaps rating them on a scale from zero to 10 or zero to 100
- monitoring symptoms of your problem in specific situations
- scheduling activities or monitoring your progress with a behavioural goal; for instance, planning or recording how many times you exercised at the gym in the past week.

SELF-MONITORING DAY BY DAY

By keeping track of problems as they occur day by day, people become more aware of the specific situations that tend to "activate" their distress. The monitoring forms used in CBT help people become more tuned in to the particular type of reactions they have to difficult situations. For instance, do certain events tend to activate feelings such as sadness, anxiety, anger, hurt or disappointment?

Monitoring forms are also used to help people become more aware of the intensity of their moods. For instance, does one situation often lead to low levels of anxiety, while another situation always leads to extremely high levels of anxiety?

Finally, monitoring forms are not just used to track problems; they are also used to help people become more aware of how well they are doing. For instance, monitoring forms can be used to rate the degree of success people have achieved toward reaching a behavioural goal, or to track their experience of pleasure or mastery (i.e., achievement and skill) during certain events and tasks.

People with depression and other emotional problems that affect motivation tend to become less involved or engaged in activities. When they do engage in an activity, they tend to report less enjoyment than they actually felt at the time they were doing the activity. One way for people to get a better idea of how they spend their days and how much pleasure and sense of mastery they derive from each activity is to keep track of what they do and how they felt at the time. If you have problems with motivation, keeping track of your activities can help you recognize that you can get more pleasure and mastery from doing things than from not doing them. In simple terms, doing things, even small things, can help you to feel better.

An activity schedule lists the days of the week across the top and the hours of the day down the left side. Your therapist may ask you to record your activities hour to hour and to make pleasure and mastery ratings on a scale from zero to 10, as seen in the example of a partially completed schedule in Table 3 below.

Table 3. Weekly activity schedule with pleasure ratings

	MONDAY	TUESDAY	WEDNESDAY
7–8 a.m.	Got up, had coffee P (pleasure) 2; M (mastery) 0	Got up, read the paper and made breakfast P 4; M 4	Got up, talked to friend overseas P 6; M 0
8–9 a.m.	Took the dog for a walk P 3; M 3	Took the dog for a walk P 2; M 3	Took the dog for a quick walk, rushed to class P 1; M 5

9–10 a.m.	Took bus to class P 0; M 4	Met study group to work on presentation P 2; M 8	Attended class P 5; M 6
10–11 a.m.	Attended class P 2; M 7	Same	Attended 2nd class P 7; M 8
11–noon		Same	Attended 3rd class P 6; M 4
noon–1 p.m.	Met friend for lunch P 6; M 1		Returned home, made healthy lunch P 4; M 7
1–2 p.m.	Attended class P 5; M 7		Caught up on laundry P 0; M 7

SELF-MONITORING SYMPTOMS

Specialized forms to help you monitor and track your symptoms throughout treatment are available for virtually all clinical problems in CBT. The process of closely monitoring and recording your experiences can in itself improve your mood and well-being, and so this is usually encouraged following the first CBT session.

If you are seeking help for anxiety, you may be asked to complete monitoring forms to record the precise symptoms of anxiety depending on the particular anxiety problem you are experiencing. For example, if you are seeking help for social anxiety, you will be asked to complete a monitoring form that will ask you to record social or performance situations in the past where you felt anxious.

If you are seeking help for obsessive-compulsive disorder, you will record the nature and distress associated with obsessive thoughts throughout the week as well as the frequency and duration of compulsive rituals.

Table 4 provides an example of a symptom monitoring form that is tailored for panic attacks. This form allows you to record all of the symptoms experienced during a panic attack over the week between sessions.

Table 4. Panic attack monitoring form

SITUATION:

Rate anxiety severity:

0	5	10
None	Moderate	Intense

Symptoms (Tick all experienced):

❏ Accelerated heart rate	❏ Dry mouth
❏ Chest pain or discomfort	❏ Inability to relax
❏ Dizziness	❏ Restlessness
❏ Paresthesia (numbness)	❏ Fatigue
❏ Trembling or shaking	❏ Discomfort
❏ Sensation of shortness of breath	❏ Sleep difficulties
❏ Blushing	❏ Irritability or anger outbursts
❏ Sweating	❏ Difficulty concentrating
❏ Nausea / growling stomach	❏ Hypervigilance for danger
❏ Muscle tension	❏ Exaggerated startle response

SCHEDULING ACTIVITIES

The same schedule used in Table 3 to monitor activities and make pleasure and mastery ratings may also be used to help you schedule. One use is to schedule activities that you may have been avoiding. This can help to remove indecisiveness around whether or not you should do an activity. For instance, if you decide in advance that you will go to the gym between 5:00 p.m. and 6:00 pm on Tuesday, you are more likely to go than if you wait to decide based on how you feel that day.

The therapist may also ask you to schedule both pleasurable activities (e.g., lunch with a friend) and mastery tasks (e.g., organizing and paying bills) for the upcoming week. You will likely also be asked to keep track of your automatic thoughts during your weekly activities to help you identify distortions or other appraisals that minimize or undermine your pleasure or sense of mastery in the activity.

A further use of the activity schedule is to help you recognize the barriers to completing tasks and to break down these tasks into smaller units to make the tasks less distressing and more likely to be accomplished. "Graded tasks" can then be constructed where you schedule the easier steps of the task before getting to more complicated and challenging parts of the task. Simply changing the structure and the approach to tasks in this way can create remarkable changes in the likelihood that you will accomplish tasks.

Exposure therapy

A standard component of CBT treatment for anxiety is exposure therapy. Exposure therapy works to reduce your fear of certain things (e.g., insects, snakes) or situations (e.g., closed spaces, heights) by gradually increasing your exposure to the feared thing or situation. To begin, you may be asked to imagine or look at pictures of that feared thing or situation (indirect exposure) and then gradually increase your exposure until you are able to touch the thing or experience the situation (direct exposure).

With gradual exposure to your fears, your anxiety decreases and you learn that your fears are excessive and irrational. This process is called habituation. Figure 1 shows that as the number of exposures to the feared thing or situation increases, the level of anxiety produced by exposure decreases.

Figure 1. Habituation curve in exposure therapy

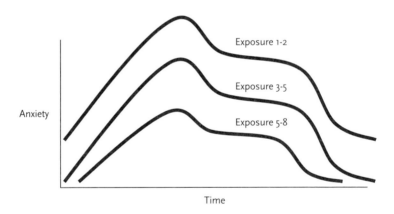

Exposure therapy usually starts with exposure to situations that create only mild-to-moderate fear and gradually progress to situations that create higher levels of anxiety. Before starting exposure therapy, you will complete a hierarchy of your fears, listing all of the situations that trigger your anxiety and the different levels of anxiety associated with each trigger. In the example of a completed hierarchy of fear in Table 5, a person who fears coming into contact with beetles rates situations involving beetles—from mildly distressing to most distressing.

Table 5. Hierarchy of feared situations: Example

FEARED SITUATION (mildly distressing to most distressing)	DISTRESS (10–100)
View cartoon drawing of beetles, then touch it	10
View photo of real beetles, then touch it	20
Stand in room with small beetles, walk within five feet of beetles	30
Walk within one foot of small beetles	40
Stand in room with large beetles, walk within five feet of beetles	50
Walk within one foot of large beetles	60
Touch small beetles with finger	70
Allow small beetles to crawl on arm	80
Touch large beetles with finger	90
Allow large beetles to crawl on arm	100

At first you will complete exposure tasks with the help of the therapist. Later, as you progress, you will be asked to do them on your own as homework between sessions. The rate at which you progress in treatment will depend on the severity of your fear and on your ability to tolerate the discomfort associated with arousing your anxiety. Exposure tasks need to be repeated and last long enough (usually not less than 30 minutes) to result in optimal improvements. You learn that anxiety comes down naturally when you remain in the fear-provoking situation long enough.

Behavioural experiments

Behavioural experiments were described on page 22 as a way of testing your underlying assumptions and beliefs. Behavioural experiments ask you to act out a feared situation to see if what you fear might happen does happen. Should the feared outcome occur, the experiments will also enable you to see how well you cope with the situation.

These tasks are behavioural because they require that you "test out" new ways of thinking by doing something differently, often by going into situations and choosing a different behavioural strategy.

5 CBT in practice: Questions and answers

Answers to frequently asked questions about CBT, such as how to find a therapist and what to expect in treatment, are outlined below.

How will I know if CBT is for me?

Most people know within the first few sessions if they are comfortable with CBT and whether it is meeting their treatment needs. The therapist will also check to see that CBT is the right "fit" for you. When the fit is not quite right, the therapist may adjust the treatment or suggest other treatment options. However, in general, CBT may be a good therapy option for you if:

• you are interested in learning practical skills to manage your present, day-to-day life and associated emotional difficulties
• you are willing and interested in practising change strategies ("homework") between sessions to consolidate improvement.

CBT may not be for you if you want to focus exclusively on past issues, if you want supportive counselling, or if you are not willing to do homework between sessions.

How can I find a qualified CBT therapist in my area?

To find the contact information for certified CBT therapists in Canada and the United States, consult the following resources:

- Academy of Cognitive Therapies
  www.academyofct.org
- Association for Behaviour and Cognitive Therapies
  www.abct.org

What can I expect on my first visit with a CBT therapist?

At your first visit, you and the CBT therapist will discuss:

- the nature and causes of your difficulties and factors that could be maintaining them
- how the therapist will apply the CBT model to your specific problems
- how the tasks that you will do in therapy can work to change different aspects of the problems
- what you want to get out of treatment
- whether CBT is a suitable treatment approach for you
- whether other treatment approaches might be called for, either instead of or in addition to CBT.

By the end of this first visit, you and the therapist will have developed a goal-oriented treatment plan to address your difficulties.

What happens in a CBT session?

CBT sessions can be given to clients individually or in groups. Both formats follow the same predictable structure, as follows:

- Mood check: The therapist asks about your mood since the previous session. This may include the use of scales to assess depression, anxiety or other emotional problems. The purpose of the mood check is to see if your mood improves from session to session.
- Bridge: The focus of the previous session is reviewed to create a bridge to the current session.
- Agenda: The therapist and client identify issues to address in the current session that will act as the agenda.
- Homework review: Homework from the previous session is reviewed to note progress and troubleshoot any difficulties that may have emerged.
- Agenda items: Agenda issues are addressed using cognitive and behavioural strategies.
- New homework: Exercises and tasks for the upcoming week are assigned.
- Summary and client feedback: Wrap up of the session.

How can I get the most out of CBT between sessions?

CBT is a treatment approach that teaches you skills to become your own therapist over time. You learn new skills in the therapy sessions, but ultimately much of the change occurs between therapy sessions when practising the skills in your own environment as part of homework. Early in treatment, the CBT therapist will suggest homework, such as monitoring thoughts and behaviours,

taking steps to reduce avoidance behaviour, conducting experiments to test out predictions and completing worksheets to challenge negative thoughts or beliefs. As treatment progresses, you
will learn to set your own homework between sessions to help you
accomplish your treatment goals. Research demonstrates that the
more you successfully practise the skills of CBT in your homework,
the better the treatment outcome.

How long does CBT last?

CBT is a time-limited, focused treatment approach. For problems
such as anxiety and depression, CBT usually involves 12 to 20 sessions. However, the length of treatment can vary, depending on the
severity and complexity of your problems—some clients improve
significantly in four to six sessions, while others may need more
than 20 sessions. Hospital-based programs targeting specific problems are usually 12 to 15 sessions.

How frequent are the sessions?

CBT usually starts out with weekly sessions. As treatment progresses, sessions may be spaced further apart, such as every two
weeks or month. Once people have finished a course of CBT, it is
common for them to return for occasional "booster" sessions to
keep up their progress, deal with any setbacks and prevent relapse
of problems. Again, hospital-based programs are typically pre-set
(e.g., a group meeting weekly at the same time for 12 weeks) and
are less flexible in terms of scheduling and spacing sessions than
community-based CBT therapists.

Do I need to prepare for CBT sessions?

Preparing to discuss a specific problem at each session helps you to get the most out of CBT. Coming prepared helps to keep you focused on your goals for therapy. It also helps to build a therapeutic relationship between you and your therapist and to communicate well throughout the session.

Will the CBT therapist be able to understand and appreciate my own unique background?

Research on CBT demonstrates that it is an effective treatment regardless of gender, race, ethnicity, culture, sexual orientation or social economic status. CBT therapists are trained to recognize the importance of cultural values and to adapt their treatments to meet culturally unique needs. They are trained, for example, to:

• be aware of their own personal values and biases and how these may influence their relationship with the client
• use skills and intervention strategies that are culturally appropriate for the person being seen
• be aware of how certain cultural processes may influence the relationship between the therapist and client.

As a client in CBT you should feel that you can openly discuss aspects of your culture or sexual orientation, for example, and that your treatment will be delivered in a manner that is consistent with these values.

Is CBT an effective treatment for children and adolescents?

CBT has been adapted for use with children and has been shown in research to be an effective intervention for a variety of clinical problems that can emerge in childhood, including anxiety and depression. The content and pacing of the therapy is adjusted to be appropriate for the child's level of development. Often, the CBT therapist will work with the parent and child—the younger the child, the more involved the parent will be in learning and delivering CBT strategies for their child's problem.

What are the common barriers that come up in CBT?

Barriers to treatment can include:

- perceived stigma associated with mental health treatment
- difficulty identifying and distinguishing emotions and their intensity
- difficulty in reflecting on thoughts
- difficulty tolerating heightened emotions
- not completing homework
- financial constraints
- chronic conditions and multiple difficulties
- low optimism toward improving
- avoiding treatment sessions.

The therapist will work with you to reduce these barriers and will also offer strategies that you can use to overcome barriers.

Should I start treatment with medications or CBT or both in combination?

Many people who seek treatment for emotional difficulties in Canada are first treated by their family doctor with one or more medications (e.g., antidepressants) before CBT is considered. Not much research has been done to show whether it is best to start treatment with medication or CBT or both. However, research has shown that CBT, with or without certain types of medications, is equally effective for the treatment of anxiety problems, and that CBT and medications together are best for treating severe depression and psychosis. Importantly, taking these kinds of medications has not been shown to interfere with CBT, and in some instances may help people to get more out of the therapy.

There is, however, one class of medication commonly prescribed to people with anxiety problems, known as benzodiazepines, which can potentially limit the benefits of CBT. Medications in this class include clonazepam (Rivotril), alprazolam (Xanax) and lorazepam (Ativan). While these medications can rapidly relieve and control anxiety in the short term, they can also make it harder to learn new things, which is essential to benefit from CBT and reduce anxiety in the long run. If you are taking these medications and are about to start CBT, your CBT therapist will want to review the advantages and disadvantages of continuing with these medications during CBT treatment.

When considering or starting CBT, discuss all of your questions or concerns about your medications with your CBT therapist and/or your prescribing medical doctor. Medications can be monitored and discussed throughout treatment and adjusted depending on your progress in CBT. Note that recommendations or changes to your medication can only be made by your prescribing doctor. If your CBT therapist is not a doctor, he or she can—with your permission—communicate with your doctor to help ensure that you receive the optimal combination of treatments.

How can I stay well after finishing CBT?

A major goal of CBT is for you to become your own therapist and to continue to practise CBT skills even after you are feeling better. You may also wish to return for follow-up or "booster" sessions from time to time. A key component of CBT treatment is teaching relapse prevention strategies. This includes helping you learn to identify the triggers and early signs of relapse and to develop an action plan to prevent downward spirals of negative emotions.

6 Alternative cognitive-behavioural approaches

Of the hundreds of psychological treatments available, several are closely related to CBT, but have distinct approaches. Although the effectiveness of these alternative CBT approaches is not as well proven as the mainstream approach described so far in this guide, the four introduced on the following pages have been found to be effective in helping people with certain types of problems. Overall, they all share a common goal of helping people learn how to "let go" of focusing on and reacting to their thoughts.

Mindfulness therapy and mindfulness-based cognitive therapy

Mindfulness techniques can be used to help people distance themselves from their negative thinking and recognize that thoughts do not have to determine behaviours. Mindfulness is a state of awareness, openness and receptiveness that allows people to engage fully in what they are doing at any given moment. Mindfulness skills are mainly taught through meditation; however, other experiential exercises (e.g., walking or eating with awareness) can also be used to teach these skills.

Mindfulness skills can be broken down into three categories:

- *Defusion*: distancing oneself from and letting go of unhelpful thoughts, beliefs and memories.
- *Acceptance*: accepting thoughts and feelings without judgment, simply allowing them to come and go rather than trying to push them out of awareness or make sense of them.
- *Contact in the present moment*: engaging fully in the here-and-now with an attitude of openness and curiosity.

Mindfulness skills promote freedom from the tendency to get drawn into automatic negative reactions to thoughts and feelings.

Mindfulness techniques have been used in the treatment of chronic pain, hypertension, heart disease, cancer, gastrointestinal disorders, eating disorders, anxiety disorders and substance use disorders. Mindfulness-based cognitive therapy has been found to be effective in reducing relapse to depression.

Acceptance and commitment therapy

While some therapies attempt to change upsetting thoughts and feelings, acceptance and commitment therapy (ACT) helps people to simply notice and accept thoughts and feelings in the present moment.

ACT views psychological suffering as being caused by avoiding or evaluating thoughts and feelings, which in turn can lead to ways of thinking that interfere with our ability to act consistently with important personal values. The focus of ACT is on helping people accept what is out of their personal control while committing to doing what is within their control to improve their quality of life.

ACT aims to help people handle the pain and stress that life inevitably brings and to create a rich, full and meaningful life. People learn how to deal with painful thoughts and feelings in ways that have less impact and influence over their lives. For example, they learn to:

• distance themselves from upsetting thoughts (cognitive defusion)
• accept experiences in the present moment
• discover important and meaningful personal values
• set goals consistent with these values
• commit to take action.

ACT has been found to be effective in treating depression, anxiety, stress, chronic pain and substance use disorders.

Dialectical behavioural therapy

Dialectical behavioural therapy (DBT) is an effective treatment for people with excessive mood swings, self-harming behaviour and other interpersonal problems related to the expression of anger.

DBT has an individual and a group component. In individual therapy, the therapist and client follow a treatment target hierarchy to guide their discussion of issues that come up between weekly sessions. First priority is given to self-harming and suicidal behaviours, then to behaviours that interfere with therapy, and next to improving the client's quality of life. The quality-of-life improvement part of the therapy involves identifying skills that the person has but is not using to full advantage, to teaching new skills, and to discussing obstacles for using those skills. Weekly group therapy focuses on acquiring new skills.

Clients keep diary cards to help monitor their use of the skills and have access to 24-hour phone consultation with their therapist.

The four modules of DBT are core mindfulness, emotion regulation (e.g., identifying and labelling emotions and reducing vulnerability to negative emotions), interpersonal effectiveness (e.g., assertiveness skills) and distress tolerance skills (e.g., crisis survival skills such as distracting, self-soothing and improving the moment).

Meta-cognitive therapy

Meta-cognitive therapy (MCT) was first developed to treat generalized anxiety disorder and is now also used to treat other anxiety disorders and depression.

Metacognition is the aspect of cognition that controls mental processes and thinking. Most people have some direct conscious experience of metacognition. For example, when a name is on the "tip of your tongue," metacognition is working to inform you that the information is somewhere in memory, even though you are unable to remember it.

People with depression or anxiety often feel as though they have lost control over their thoughts and behaviours. Their thinking and attention become fixed in patterns of brooding and dwelling on themselves and on threatening information. They develop coping behaviours that they believe are helpful, but that can actually worsen and prolong emotional distress. This pattern of thinking is called cognitive-attentional syndrome (CAS).

In MCT, people learn to reduce the CAS by developing new ways of controlling their thinking and attention and of relating to depressive or anxious thoughts and beliefs. They also learn to modify the beliefs that give rise to the CAS.

References

Burns, D.D. (1999). *The Feeling Good Handbook: The New Mood Therapy.* New York: HarperCollins.

Resources

Hundreds of self-help and professional books on CBT are available. Listed below are a few examples. Many of the web links listed later in this section provide an even broader list of reading and workbook options.

CBT self-help books for anxiety and depression

ANXIETY DISORDERS (ADULTS)

Antony, M.M. & Norton, P.J. (2009). *The Anti-Anxiety Workbook: Proven Strategies to Overcome Worry, Panic, Phobias, and Obsessions.* New York: Guilford Press.

Bourne, E.J. (2003). *Coping with Anxiety: 10 Simple Ways to Relieve Anxiety, Fear & Worry.* Oakland, CA: New Harbinger.

ANXIETY DISORDERS (CHILDREN)

Rapee, R.M., Spence, S.H., Cobham, V., Wignall, A. & Lyneham, H. (2008). *Helping your Anxious Child: A Step-by-Step Guide for Parents, 2nd ed.* Oakland, CA: New Harbinger.

DEPRESSION

Greenberger, D. & Padesky, C.A. (1995). *Mind Over Mood: Change How You Feel by Changing the Way You Think.* New York: Guilford Press.

Knaus, B.J. (2006). *The Cognitive Behavioral Workbook for Depression: A Step-by-Step Program*. Oakland, CA: New Harbinger.

GENERAL ANXIETY DISORDER

Craske, M.G. & Barlow, D.H. (2006). *Mastery of Your Anxiety and Worry (*2nd ed.). New York: Oxford. (See also accompanying therapist manual.)

Meares, K. & Freeston, M. (2008). *Overcoming Worry: A Self-Help Guide Using Cognitive Behavioral Techniques*. New York: Basic Books.

OBSESSIVE-COMPULSIVE DISORDER

Abramowitz, J.S. (2009). *Getting over OCD: A 10-Step Workbook for Taking Back Your Life*. New York: Guilford Press.

Hyman, B.M. & Pedrick, C. (2005). *The OCD Workbook: Your Guide to Breaking Free from Obsessive-Compulsive Disorder (*2nd ed.). Oakland, CA: New Harbinger.

PANIC DISORDER

Antony, M.M. & McCabe, R.E. (2004). *10 Simple Solutions to Panic: How to Overcome Panic Attacks, Calm Physical Symptoms, and Reclaim Your Life*. Oakland, CA: New Harbinger.

Wilson, R. (2009). *Don't Panic: Taking Control of Anxiety Attacks (*3rd ed.). New York: HarperCollins.

POSTTRAUMATIC STRESS DISORDER

Rothbaum, B.O., Foa, E.B. & Hembree, E.A. (2007). *Reclaiming Your Life from a Traumatic Experience* (Workbook). New York: Oxford. (See also accompanying therapist manual.)

SOCIAL ANXIETY DISORDER

Markway, B.G., Pollard, C.A., Flynn, T. & Carmin, C.N. (1992). *Dying of Embarrassment: Help for Social Anxiety and Phobia.* New York: New Harbinger.

Stein, M.B. & Walker, J.R. (2009). *Triumph over Shyness: Conquering Social Anxiety Disorder* (2nd ed.). Silver Spring, MD: Anxiety Disorders Association of America.

CBT self-help books for other disorders

ATTENTION DEFICIT DISORDER

Safren, S.A., Sprich, S., Perlman, C.A. & Otto, M.W. (2005). *Mastering Your Adult ADHD: Client Workbook. A Cognitive-Behavioral Treatment Program.* New York: Oxford University Press. (See also accompanying therapist manual.)

BODY DYSMORPHIC DISORDER

Claiborn, J. & Pedrick, C. (2002). *The BDD Workbook: Overcome Body Dysmorphic Disorder and End Body Image Obsessions.* Oakland, CA: New Harbinger.

BODY-FOCUSED IMPULSIVE DISORDERS

Franklin, M.E. & Tolin, D.F. (2007). *Treating Trichotillomania: Cognitive-Behavioral Therapy for Hair Pulling and Related Problems.* New York: Springer.

EATING DISORDERS

McCabe, R.E., McFarlane, T.L. & Olmstead, M.P. (2004). *Overcoming Bulimia: Your Comprehensive, Step-By-Step Guide to Recovery.* Oakland, CA: New Harbinger.

HYPOCHONDRIASIS AND HEALTH ANXIETY

Asmundson, G.J.G. & Taylor, S. (2005). *It's Not All In Your Head: How Worrying About Your Health Could Be Making You Sick – and What You Can Do About It.* New York: Guilford.

SCHIZOPHRENIA

Beck, A.T., Rector, N.A., Stolar, N. & Grant, P. (2008). *Schizophrenia: Cognitive Theory, Research, and Therapy.* New York: Guilford Press.

SLEEP DISORDERS

Edinger, J.D. & Carney, C.E. (2008). *Overcoming Insomnia: A Cognitive-Behavioral Therapy Approach Workbook.* New York: Oxford University Press. (See also accompanying therapist manual).

SUBSTANCE USE DISORDER

Daley, D.C. & Marlatt, D.C. (2006). *Overcoming Your Alcohol or Drug Problem: Effective Recovery Strategies* (2nd ed.). New York: Oxford University Press. (See also accompanying therapist manual.)

CBT WITH DIVERSE POPULATIONS

Hays, P. & Iwamasa, G. (Eds.). (2006). *Culturally Responsive Cognitive-Behavioral Therapy: Assessment, Practice, and Supervision.* Washington, DC: American Psychological Association Press.

Internet resources

Academy of Cognitive Therapy
www.academyofct.org

American Psychiatric Association
www.psych.org

American Psychological Association
www.apa.org
(Click "Psychology Topics," then "A-Z Topics," then "Therapy.")

Association for Behavioral and Cognitive Therapies
www.abct.org

Canadian Mental Health Association
www.cmha.ca

Centre for Addiction and Mental Health
www.camh.net

Counselling Resource
http://counsellingresource.com

Royal College of Psychiatrists
www.rcpsych.ac.uk/default.aspx
(Click "Mental Health Info," then "Treatments," then "CBT.")